INTRODUCTION

In the same way as other enhancements, berberine is gotten from plants. "Berberine is a kind of substance compound called an alkaloid that is tracked down in the roots, leaves, stems, and barks of plants, like barberry, Oregon grape, and tree turmeric," says Vicki Shanta Retelny, RDN, the Chicago-based creator of The Fundamental Manual for

Sound Mending Food varieties.

Enrolled dietitians ordinarily recommend "eating your nutrients" as food (particularly products of the soil), yet that is precarious to do with berberine, and not as a result of the yellow compound's unpleasant taste. "Berberine can be consumed through these plants, however they are unprecedented in the US," says Davis. "Berberine is considerably more open

through a supplemental structure."

QUICK TALK

Berberine is a somewhat new expansion to the enhancement world, yet you might have known about it being alluded to on TikTok and other virtual entertainment as "nature's Ozempic." This reference is a sign of approval for the diabetes drug that has overwhelmed the world, principally due to its infamous weight reduction incidental effects.

As an enhancement, the buzz around berberine fundamentally connects with its utility as a characteristic guide for individuals with type 2 diabetes, elevated cholesterol, or hypertension. MedlinePlus notes it could try and fortify the heartbeat, possibly assisting individuals with specific heart conditions. (Note: Pregnant and breastfeeding ladies, babies, and youngsters shouldn't take berberine.)

Despite the fact that berberine has as of late been at the center of attention, it has a long history of restorative use. "Berberine is a compound tracked down normally in specific plants," makes sense of Mascha Davis, RDN, a Los Angeles-based enrolled dietitian-nutritionist and the creator of Eat Your Nutrients. "It has been utilized for a really long time in conventional Chinese medication." As per Remembrance Sloan

Kettering, berberine has been taken in the past to treat contaminations, as well as to help stomach related conditions and fiery issues.

Anyway, does berberine merit its standing as "nature's Ozempic?" Could it at any point assist with directing glucose or help weight reduction, and above all, is it safe? Find more about berberine and whether you should converse with your primary care physician about the enhancement, or take a pass.

utilizes

There are various justifications for why individuals could begin taking berberine (yet it's vital to converse with your doctor before you take any enhancement). For instance, Nebraska Medication specifies guarantees that berberine may assist with elevated cholesterol and hypertension, as well as individuals with type 2 diabetes.

HERE IS THE FULL RUNDOWN OF EXPECTED USES OF BERBERINE

•May assist individuals with type 2 diabetes bring down their glucose levels

•Could assist with bringing down high "awful" LDL cholesterol levels and fatty substance levels

•Could assist with lessening pulse levels

•May assist with facilitating blister in the mouth (when applied in a gel structure)

•Could assist individuals with polycystic ovarian disorder (or PCOS)

SYMPTOMS OF BERBERINE

While symptoms of berberine are moderately remarkable, a few clinical preliminaries make revealed gentle gastrointestinal side impacts, including

Xu X, Yi H, Wu J, et al. Restorative impact of berberine on metabolic infections: Both pharmacological information and clinical proof. Biomedicine

- Loss of hunger

- Sickness

- Retching

- Stomach torment

- Stoppage

- The runs

- Gas

The vast majority of these aftereffects appear to determine inside the initial a month of purpose.

DOSAGE OF BERBERINE

there is no settled measurements for berberine supplements. Nonetheless, most investigations have shown benefits with dosages somewhere in the range of 0.4 and 2 g each day, taken for up to two years

Further examination is expected to decide the ideal for different ailments.

Chat with your medical services supplier prior to taking berberine to guarantee that the enhancement and measurements are proper for your particular necessities.

STEP BY STEP INSTRUCTIONS TO TAKE BERBERINE

Berberine isn't tracked down in ordinary food sources, so you should take an enhancement if you have any desire to add it to your eating routine.

Berberine supplements are sold in different structures, including containers, tablets, fluid, and powder. Albeit more uncommon, berberine can likewise be found in effective gels and eye drops. Berberine enhancements can be bought in wellbeing food stores, pharmacies, or on the web.

There are no authority proposals on the most proficient method to take berberine. Notwithstanding, most makers suggest isolating the everyday portion of berberine into three more modest dosages, taken before feasts.

When taken as suggested, it might require a little while to

a while to see medical advantages.

IS BERBERINE SAFE?

Berberine is by and large very much endured with a decent wellbeing profile. It is viewed as safe for most solid grown-ups when utilized topically and taken in dosages of up to 1.5g everyday for six months.

Berberine is believed to be dangerous during pregnancy, as it might cross the placenta and damage the creating baby. Berberine is likewise not suggested while breastfeeding in light of the fact that it could be moved to the baby through bosom milk.19

In babies, berberine may cause jaundice (yellowing of the skin) and lead to a kind of cerebrum harm called kernicterus

There aren't an adequate number of studies to decide the security of berberine in kids.

MEDICATION COLLABORATIONS

While research is restricted, berberine may cooperate with the accompanying medications:19

• Cyclosporine (Neoral, Sandimmune): Berberine might diminish how rapidly the body separates cyclosporine (a prescription that lessens insusceptible reaction), expanding its secondary effects.

•Diabetes Berberine might diminish your glucose levels. When joined with diabetes prescriptions, it might cause your glucose to drop excessively low.

•Pulse meds: Since berberine may bring down circulatory strain, joining it with circulatory strain meds might cause a hazardous drop in pulse.

•Robitussin DM (Dextromethorphan): Berberine might diminish

your body's capacity to separate dextromethorphan, expanding its belongings and incidental effects.

•Blood thinners: Berberine might slow blood thickening. Taking it close by blood thinners might expand the gamble of swelling and dying.

Berberine likewise can possibly associate with spices and different enhancements that influence blood coagulating, glucose levels, or circulatory strain.

Berberine doesn't seem to cooperate with any food varieties.

On the off chance that you take physician endorsed drugs or dietary enhancements, talk with your medical care supplier to guarantee no potential cooperations happen

Might You at any point Take An excessive amount of Berberine?

While berberine is for the most part thought to be protected, taking an excess of

may build the gamble of
incidental effects and security
concerns.

CONCLUSION

In the event that you're actually considering berberine, it's critical to get your doctor's close down first. "Make a point to talk with your primary care physician and dietitian prior to taking berberine to check whether it very well may be ideal for you," prompts Davis.

For individuals with type 2 diabetes, coronary illness, and conditions like PCOS, berberine could give benefits.

"Berberine, alongside legitimate eating routine and way of life changes, can be helpful for treating specific circumstances and could be a phenomenal option to your enhancements," Davis adds. All things considered, there are secondary effects to know about, similar to stomachaches. Kids and children, as well as pregnant and breastfeeding ladies, shouldn't take berberine supplements. Individuals who take specific meds ought to converse with their PCP first prior to attempting it.